THE DAVID HUME INSTITUTE

HOW SHOULD HEALTH SERVICES BE FINANCED?

THE DAVID HUME INSTITUTE

How Should Health Services Be Financed?

A PATIENT'S VIEW

Allan Massie

Report on a Conference organised by The David Hume Institute
and Royal College of Physicians, Edinburgh held on 10 June 1988

ABERDEEN UNIVERSITY PRESS

First published 1988
Aberdeen University Press
A member of the Pergamon Group

© The David Hume Institute 1988

British Library Cataloguing in Publication Data

Massie, Alan
  How should health services be financed? : a
  patient's view.
  1. Health services. Financing
  I. Title   II. David Hume Institute
  338.4′33621

  ISBN 0-08-036585-X

Printed in Great Britain
The University Press
Aberdeen

Contents

Foreword

In the early spring of this year, as the crescendo of parliamentary debate on funding the National Health Service became more deafening, The David Hume Institute and the Royal College of Physicians, Edinburgh agreed to mount a conference to discuss the basic issues of financing health services. The debate on this, as on most public issues, centres on London where the attitudes and experience of those living in the southeast predominate. The Devil may have all the best tunes but he should not be allowed to monopolise the best orchestras too. In Scotland there is a tradition of excellence in Medicine and Political Economy. The conference brought leading practitioners in both disciplines into an ensemble to hear and develop each others views and to share them with an informed audience in the splendid setting of the Royal College of Physicians' conference suite in Queen Street, Edinburgh. The names of the Speakers and Discussants are listed on page 51. With the help of many people in the professional bodies, the universities, the Regional Health Boards, Local and Central Government, it was possible to bring together an audience whose distinction matched that of the Speakers and Discussants.

But who is the object of all this high-level analysis and discussion? It is that inveterate absentee at conferences, the common man, rich or poor, in the waiting room or the ward bed. The usual outcome of a conference is a list of evanescent resolutions with an edited version of the papers presented and the discussion which, in David Hume's phrase, falls dead-born from the press. Instead, Allan Massie was asked to represent the patient public and to write up his reactions to the day's proceedings. He has produced a critique which is short, shrewd and very elegant. Anyone with political, professional or administrative responsibility for the provision of health services who seeks a lucid expression of the highest common factor of public opinion on the subject will find it here.

It goes without saying that Allan Massie's views are his own. The David Hume Institute has no collective view on this or any other public issue but is strongly committed to rational enquiry into them.

The David Hume Institute
16 Hope Street,
Charlotte Square,
Edinburgh
9 August 1988

Acknowledgements

The David Hume Institute gratefully acknowledges the financial support offered by the following organisations which made possible both the Conference and the publication of this report:

The Esmée Fairbairn Trust
King Edward's Hospital Fund for London
The Nuffield Provincial Hospitals Trust

The Institute also wishes to thank the Royal College of Physicians, Edinburgh for the use of its conference facilities and for administrative help.

Biographical Note

Allan Massie has been described as Scotland's finest living novelist, and works such as *The Death of Men* and *Augustus* have received wide acclaim. He also writes regularly on political affairs in the *Sunday Times*. This is his second contribution to The David Hume Institute, the first being his lecture on *The Novelist's View of the Market Economy* (Hume Occasional Paper No. 7).

I Paying for Health

1.   This paper arises from a Conference held by The David Hume Institute and the Royal College of Physicians, Edinburgh on 10 June 1988. Its title was: 'How Should Health Services Be Financed?'. Inevitably the discussion was wider than this might suggest, questions of financing developing into arguments about organisation. Moreover it was, as it must always be, impossible to pursue these questions without also considering the nature of health services and the philosophy which animates them. Finally, this philosophy may itself be separated into two elements: political and moral.

2.   I propose in this introduction to offer some general observations under these headings, and to do so in reverse order. I shall therefore start by considering the moral philosphy of health and conclude by commenting on questions of finance. This method has the advantage of putting the horse before the cart because it is the moral philosophy which pulls the health service wagon.

3.   In the second part of the paper I shall offer a critical report of the arguments advanced by the various speakers and some of the responses from the floor. Finally, I shall attempt to offer a judgement of the merits of these arguments.

4.   I claim no special knowledge of these matters. That is both the strength and weakness of my position. It is weak because anything I say can probably be challenged by an expert producing evidence of which I am ignorant. But it is strong because I have no prior or professional commitment to any particular point of view. Moreover, as a layman, I am also a prospective patient, one who will be the beneficiary or victim of the professionals' skill or lack of skill, intelligent organisation or administrative ineptitude. I may be disinterested where the argument is concerned, but I have, like more than 55 million others, a clear interest in the results of these arguments.

II   The Moral Philosophy of Health Services

5.   'Illness of any kind is hardly a thing to be encouraged in others. Health is the primary duty of life.' So said Lady Bracknell in *The Importance of Being Earnest*. She added that she did not 'in any way approve of the modern sympathy with invalids', and when one hears economists talk of certain methods of health care encouraging 'excessive consumption', it may seem that some modern theorists agree with her. So indeed do those General Practitioners who would welcome the imposition of modest, if recoverable, charges which would discourage frivolous or unnecessary demands on their time.

6.   This then may be taken as a convenient expression of the philosphy that informs the provision of medicine: 'health is the primary duty of life.' Many of us would agree with her that it is more important to discourage illness in others than in ourselves. People loth to consult a doctor are often quick to tell others to do so. I mention this now because there was at the Conference much talk of 'the patient as consumer', and it occurs to me that he or she is often driven to consume by family or friends rather than inclination. Most of us do not really consume health care, which is a vile phrase, as we consume food and drink. We do not go to hospital as willingly as we go on holiday. If we are indeed consumers, we are also reluctant ones. Indeed the patient may be an involuntary consumer, who consumes in an unconscious condition. This is not a frivolous distinction; it is more frivolous to pretend that it does not exist.

7.   Good health is desirable, but it is hard to compare it with other desirable objects, such as a house, a motor-car, a holiday, a cigar or a bottle of wine. This is not only because in our present system there is for most of us no price-tag attached. It would be perfectly possible to put a price on the provision of any medical service, and it would still be felt to be of a different order, for we find it difficult to dissociate the idea of health from life itself. We know of course that people can live in miserable ill-health. That is not the point, which is rather that the condition of health is ineluctably part of the condition of living. Health is like sunshine; we mostly want as much of it as we can get. We recognise its value, but we find it hard to price.

8.   It is not only the patient who experiences this difficulty. Doctors are themselves in the position of the mediaeval king who found himself compelled to agree that he would deny justice to no man. Though some speakers talked of patients being denied treatment on account of 'clinical judgement', it is nevertheless widely believed that doctors may not deny health to their patients. It is their duty to do what is possible to alleviate pain and cure illness and disease. We may accept that a banker should say that he has no interest in a particular account, but we think it would be unethical for a doctor to rebuff a patient in like manner.

9.   Yet, when Lady Bracknell said that 'health is the primary duty of life', she was being confoundedly modern. Earlier ages would not have agreed; or rather, they might have prefaced the noun 'health' with the adjective 'spiritual'. Our concern with bodily and mental health has grown more urgent as our belief in personal immortality has withered. Medicine has supplanted theology, and in our secular society the highest good is represented by health. It is astonishing to reflect that in the United States in 1985 10.8 per cent of the Gross Domestic product was expended on health care; this represented 1,776 dollars for each person in the country. In the age of religion the Church used to demand a tithe of the faithful's income; and now the health services do.

10.   It may be observed that the Christian tradition in these matters has always been ambiguous. Jesus himself performed miracles of healing, and in the nineteenth century people were so impressed by these that the Church of Jesus Christ Scientist was established, one of the most durable examples of alternative medicine. Nevertheless, despite this, and despite a long history of charitable religious foundations which occupied themselves with the care of the sick, the Christian Church has concerned itself more with the care of souls than the care of bodies. Now the development of medical science coinciding with the decay of religion has shifted the balance. A concern with spiritual health may still manifest itself in the new guise of psychotherapy, and the proliferation of mental hospitals, psychiatric units and such like bears witness to the importance of spiritual health and also represents one of the chief costs of any health service; nevertheless in our time we have relocated the Kingdom of Heaven. It is here on earth and is represented by good health. We may say of health what Dr Johnson said of Greek: that every man gets as much of it as he can.

11.   Yet even this is not quite true. Most of us neglect our health most of the time. We eat what we are told not to eat. We drink too much. We smoke cigarettes. We inject ourselves with drugs. We don't take enough exercise. Preventive medicine receives lip-honour only, and we prefer the gratification of the instant to the good we choose to ignore. Flagrant disregard for health is common, and this must be set against the evidence to the contrary which also abounds: offered by the followers of diets, the joggers, the aerobic dances, and the anxious folk who flock to their doctor's surgery. Nevertheless even those who neglect their health may find themselves echoing St Augustine who prayed 'oh Lord, make me chaste, but not yet'.

12.   So Lady Bracknell was right. Her dictum is today's creed. It expresses the moral philosophy of health. The old public school precept— *mens sana in corpore sano*—has become the individual and national watchword. It is what we aim to achieve.

III   The Political Philosophy of Health Services

13.   If the moral philosophy of Health services is a modern idea, so is the corresponding political philosophy. Of course States have long applied certain regulations concerning health. They have responded to epidemics by passing measures about sanitation, and have undertaken public works for sanitary purposes. Beyond that, however, health care was till recently a private matter, the responsibility either of individuals or of charitable bodies. The idea that the State should make itself responsible for caring for the health of its citizens is hardly more than half-a-century old in this country. It is younger even than that in the USA. The socialisation of medicine is a post-war development, but it is one which could not be reversed now. All the plans for the reform of the National Health Service start with the assumption that it is the duty of the State to secure, and probably provide, a certain quantity of health care; no one disputes that the cost of providing health services for people who are too poor to pay for them themselves should be borne by the public purse.

14.   It is important to be clear about this, because there are two corollaries: the existence of the National Health Service is the consequence of poverty; and the obstacle to the reform of that service is the persistence of poverty. One other point may be made in this connection. Though economists or sociologists may determine a 'poverty line' below which people are classed as poor, common sense assures us that there are gradations of poverty. People above that imaginary line can afford some things, but not others: they might be able to pay a visiting fee to a doctor, but unable to pay for major surgery. If we are considering insurance, we might remember that some people can afford to insure a small family saloon, but could not afford to insure a Rolls-Royce.

15.   Health care is expensive, but if everyone could afford it, the State could be left out of the relationship between patients, doctors and hospitals. Unfortunately it is beyond the resources of many, and such as cannot provide for themselves, either by direct payments or by means of an insurance policy, are frequently those who need it most. No matter what reforms in the financing of the NHS might be effected, there would still remain several million people who must either have their health care financed by the State, in one mode or other, or go without. That is the ineluctable consequence of poverty. If it were not for the poor, we might leave the provision of health care to the market; but to do so would inflict another degree of impoverishment on those who are poor already. It is then the poor who make a national health service necessary, and the gradations of poverty which make any reform complicated and hazardous.

16.   The principle on which our NHS was established was that its services should be free at the point of use. This has been trimmed at the edges by the imposition of certain charges, but it remains central. It is not of course beyond challenge, and much of the current debate is the result of such challenge. This is, as we shall see, at its most formidable when the argument is shifted away from principle and towards questions of efficiency. Conversely it is most vigorously resisted on philosophical grounds.

17. That is to say, the defence of the status quo rests on the principle that income should not determine the quality of service provided to anyone: that the poorest should get as good a deal as the richest; that the pauper will be treated with the same skill and given the same quantity of the same quality of attention as the millionaire.

18. It is then a principle that levels of income, which determine so much in life, should determine nothing in matters of health. The justification of this political philosophy is the moral philosophy outlined earlier: the conviction that health is the highest good which should be denied to none. Therefore the provision of health services is placed in a quite separate category from other provisions. No one disputes that the millionaire may eat foie gras while the down-and-out makes good with soup kitchens. No one disputes that he may live in a bigger and finer house, and we do not demand that municipally supplied housing should be as good as that which is available to buy; but we do expect the general practitioner to give as careful attention to a poor man as to a rich man, and if the millionaire and the down-and-out both collapse in the street, we expect them to be given the same emergency care in the same hospital by the same doctors.

19. The provision of Health care is, therefore, the one area in which, notwithstanding the existence of parallel private systems of health care, egalitarianism is believed to have triumphed. Therefore no reform of the National Health Service will be popular unless it is believed to guarantee the right of equal access to rich and poor.

IV   The Nature of Health Services

20. The most striking feature of health care is its variety. This is so evident that it is easily ignored. Yet it is the sort of commonplace which becomes more remarkable the longer you think of it. We are frequently told that the National Health Service is the largest employer in Europe, and it is easy to think of it as a monolithic organisation, and to talk of it as such. But it is nothing of the kind, and indeed the principal obstacle to clear thinking about the NHS and its problems may be the idea of the National

Health Service as such; for this leads the unwary to suppose that there is indeed such an entity which can be usefully so described. In reality of course it is fragmented geographically and functionally, and the nature of its problems reflects these divisions. The problem of providing satisfactory health care is not the same in the Highlands of Scotland as in Central London.

21.   This habit of thought which ignores the variety of health services has an unfortunate consequence. If you think of the NHS as an entity, this being a species of abstract construction, then you can think in terms of problems and solutions. If on the other hand you realise that you are talking about the myriad of independent acts which represent the continuing provision of health care, then it is clear that talk of solutions is irrelevant and misleading. The provision of health services is susceptible of improvement, but never of solution. Mathematics enter the argument, but health care is not a problem in mathematics.

22.   The first distinction is between what is called 'primary' and what is called 'secondary' health care. In common language this means the difference between the work of general practitioners and the work of hospitals. In this country a patient will first, except in cases of emergency, report to his or her GP who may choose to refer the matter to a hospital.

23.   That is a clear pattern but within it are to be found many different varieties of care. The patient may visit the doctor, or the doctor may call on the patient. This variation imposes different demands on each. In the first case the patient will have to spend time in travelling and probably in waiting. In the second it is the doctor who travels, thus spending part of the working day performing no medical function. If the test of the doctor's efficiency is merely the number of patients seen in a day, when it is most efficient to collect as many as possible in his surgery or health centre. This is all the more true because many of the demands on his time will be frivolous in the sense that examination fails to discover any ailment. But of course such an attempt to determine a doctor's worth in quantifable terms is inadequate: a visit to a housebound old lady may be more beneficial to that patient than fifteen routine examinations are to others. Moreover, an examination may be beneficial even if it reveals that the patient has nothing wrong. The mere experience of conversation with the doctor may be valuable.

24.   To say this is to state the obvious, but the obvious is worth stating because it may remind us that while we can devise a system of pricing a doctor's work, we have no objective means of assessing its value. The incompatibility of price and value is at the heart of the Health Service debate. It is this incompatibility which makes it so difficult to cost medical work. It is impossible to construct an equation which will make the identifiable costs of treating a child with meningitis equal the value of that work.

25.   I should like to pursue this in a short digression. Let us suppose there are two patients with a similar heart condition. Each is thought to require an operation to have an approximately equal chance of surviving it. Both operations are performed: Patient A comes through, B dies. Now it is possible to establish the cost of the operations (in rather crude terms). One can therefore say that the value of the operation was great for A, and anything but that for B. One might even, considering the costs, say it was worthwhile for A but not for B. But these conclusions could not have been reached before the operation. The value for both then was imponderable. And if B had survived six months or a year, would that have altered one's judgement? The fact is that cost (or price) is objective; value subjective.

26.   In the category of secondary health care, there is equal variety. A patient may visit a hospital to make use of out-patient facilities, or be accommodated in a hospital bed. Here again the patient's experience will vary, and the imposition of costs will be different accordingly. He or she may suffer greater inconvenience as an out-patient, and, in doing so, cause less trouble to the hospital staff and impose lower costs on the hospital. It is common in many hospitals for a number of patients to be given appointments at the same time. This ensures that the medical staff's time will not be wasted, and, unfortunately, that the patient's will. It is interesting to compare the system by which dentists allocate their time. In general they adhere to timetables, and patients who have made appointments individually are not accustomed to have to wait long after the appointed time for treatment. I mention this here because it is such matters as the apparent indifference to the inconvenience caused to patients by hospitals' administrative routine which have led critics to describe the service as 'producer-oriented'. It is a relevant point of course that is much easier to change your dentist than your hospital.

27.   Among in-patients, differences are equally marked: some require surgery, others do not. Surgical treatment is divided into acute surgery, which is generally urgent, and non-acute surgery, some varieties of which are described as 'elective'. Other patients require only treatment and nursing. Yet another division exists between those who are in hospital to be cured, and those who can only be cared for. Even these categories can overlap. Then our hospitals also assume responsibility for a variety of people who, for different reasons such as alcoholism, drug-addiction, psychiatric disorders, or senility, are incapable of functioning as normal social beings or of managing their own lives. The condition of some of these patients may improve sufficiently to enable them to live out of hospital again; the condition of others can only deteriorate.

28.   When we are talking of finance and payment, it is evident that a great gulf exists between those patients who will resume a normal life in which they are capable of earning money, and those who will not.

29.   Nor does variety end there. The development of preventive medicine, especially scanning, has added yet another dimension to medical care. In some cases it has improved the quality of that care while increasing the cost; this is because the great majority of scans reveal the patient to be in good health and therefore in no need of further treatment. A cost has therefore been incurred to establish that there is no need of medical intervention. In other cases the scan may avert expensive treatment by making it possible for a condition to be dealt with earlier and more cheaply.

30.   One further general observation about the nature of health care may be useful. It is an exercise in collaborration, first between doctor and patient, then between different branches of the medical profession, then between the doctors and the hospital administrators, finally between the medical staff and the ancillary workers. All share a common aim. Yet at the same time all these examples of collaboration may also involve conflict. We may observe a conflict of interest, a conflict of priorities, even a conflict of language. Finally, a great many of the acts which in sum represent the care of even one person's health cannot be reasonably or intelligently costed.

V   The Organisation of Health Services

31.   The National Health Service was neither conceived in the abstract nor created out of nothing. It was, rather, imposed on what already existed, and this had grown up, haphazardly, over a long period of time, without coherent system and according to no general plan.

32.   Though it is unlikely that any Health Service conceived as a unity would bear much resemblance to that which we have, the present reality should not be disparaged for that reason. On the contrary, it has certain obvious virtues, the chief of which is that everything in it—each hospital or doctor's surgery for example—was established where it is in response to perceived needs or opportunities. Nevertheless the result was that the National Health Service inherited a pattern of hospitals in which where was both duplication and fragmentation of resources, a situation which, however suited to the public who used those hospitals, has come to seem less and less justifiable as medical technology has grown ever more complicated and expensive. Many of the present troubles of the NHS are a consequence of its successes; the advance of medicine has increased the demands made of the service.

33.   The development of maternity units may be used to illustrate some of the consequences of the advance of medical science. Births used to take place either at home or in local cottage hospitals. Now they generally take place in large hospitals which possess the most up-to-date facilities for post-natal care. These facilities are expensive, and it is hard on economic grounds to justify their duplication in smaller hospitals. This may mean that a better (and safer) medical service is provided at the expense of a poorer social service. At present for instance argument is going on in the North-East of Scotland about proposals put forward by Grampian Health Board to close the maternity wards at a number of smaller outlying hospitals and to concentrate this activity in Aberdeen. There may well be medical advantages, and there are certainly economic advantages, in this proposal. On the other hand, it will make visiting a mother and baby in hospital more difficult and more expensive for other members of the family. When a birth is straightforward, with no complications, the service to the patient and her family will be poorer, or at least less satisfactory.

34. The expectation of a higher standard of medical care must be met. At the same time it has seemed necessary to try to check the rising cost of such care. Recent administrative reforms have had this dual intention. The introduction of managerial techniques recommended in the Griffiths Report was intended to facilitate collaboration between different elements of the service, and to improve efficiency. Co-ordination and collaboration, it is suggested, need not exclude competition; hence the opening of ancillary services to tender, the proposals for an internal market to operate between different hospitals and different Health Boards, and the suggestion of collaborative competition with the private sector.

35. To some this has always existed. The NHS was founded on a compromise which permitted consultants to retain private patients and to accommodate them in pay-beds or private wards within NHS hospitals. In the late 1970s one response to pressures on the NHS seemed to be to squeeze out the private sector and effect a complete separation between it and the NHS; this was favoured by some of the unions and by Left-inclining opinion. Now the wheel has turned, and the argument runs that both public and private medicine can benefit from closer association which will result in co-operation and competition being simultaneously pursued.

36. Nothing has been more remarkable than the increase in the numbers of administrative staff, which has taken place in all sectors of the service. Forty years ago many family doctors worked without secretarial assistance, or with part-time unpaid help provided by their wives. Now the group practices which have become the norm invariably employ several secretaries/receptionists. No doubt it would be impossible for them to function otherwise. Yet here, at a basic level, we have an example of what seems to be a general rule: the search for greater medical efficiency leads to higher administrative costs. This is even more evident at hospital and Health Board levels. The general managers, who were introduced to try to bring coherence to the system and to control costs, may have had some success; but they themselves represent another layer of costly bureaucracy. They may not yet have had time to prove themselves, but there is no persuasive evidence that they have achieved greater medical efficiency. Critics, who include doctors, fear that the higher administrative costs must in time impair the efficiency which is sought.

37. The organisation of the NHS makes a timid bow to democratic principles in England and Wales, where a number of Health Board members are nominated by local government councils, and none in Scotland, where all are appointed by the Secretary of State. In fact the position is not so very different since his appointees invariably include regional and district councillors. The powers of Health Boards are great, but their autonomy is limited by both statutory requirements and financial constraints. They have no responsibility for raising the money they spend, and they are subject to the overriding authority of the department of Health and Social Security or, in Scotland, the Secretary of State. Their principal functions are planning, administration and the co-ordination of diverse activities, though planning of capital investment remains the responsibility of central government.

38.   Any questioning of the structure of the NHS might well start with the examination of how Health Boards work. They represent the interests of neither the consumer nor the producer. Instead they may be taken as the guardians of a less distinct interest: that of Society as a whole. It is perhaps however even more reasonable to question the role of central government, and this means first of all questioning the means by which we have chosen to finance the Health Service.

VI   The Financing of Health Services

39.   If I say comparatively little about this here, it is because this was the nominal subject of the Conference, though, as will be seen, some of the papers delivered ranged more widely.

40.   The NHS has always been financed almost entirely out of taxation. We pay no health tax, as such, because, with one or two minor exceptions such as the Road Fund Licence and the Radio and Television Licence, it has not been customary in Britain to allocate particular taxes to particular purposes. The money for the Health Service comes therefore from General Taxation, and the amount allocated to the NHS in each financial year is determined as a result of submissions from the ministries concerned (the DHSS and the Scottish Office) to the Treasury, and subsequent discussions between the Treasury and those ministries, ultimately at ministerial level. The NHS therefore competes with other objects of public expenditure for a share of the government's income, and the amount of money spent on the Health Service can never be determined solely by what the responsible ministries think it necessary or desirable to spend. The money available is the result of a compromise between the Treasury and all spending ministries, but even before that point is reached, it is determined also by the Government's view as to the proper level of public expenditure expressed as a share of the Gross National Product, and also by its view of the morality of rates of tax. For most of the history of the NHS, Governments have been committed to high public spending and have had no objection to high rates of personal taxation, or none at least which went beyond considerations of electoral disadvantage. Recently however we have had a Government of a different complexion, which wishes to reduce Public Expenditure as a share of GDP, and regards high rates of income tax as morally indefensible. Nevertheless, despite this ideological commitment, spending on the NHS has risen very considerably in real terms under this Government.

41.   It is not of course necessary to finance a National Health Service in this way. There are some who would like to see specific sums of money raised for health spending by means of an identifiable health tax. They believe that this would enable the consumer to choose between higher and lower levels of spending on the NHS in full consciousness that this would affect his or her own disposable income. It must be doubtful if this would be so. Certainly it is hard to visualise a political party entering a General Election with the promise to lower the Health Service tax.

42.   Another proposal is that the Health Service should continue to be financed out of general taxation, but that people might be allowed to contract out; to do so, they would take out private health insurance policies, and if they wished to be treated in a NHS hospital, their insurance company would be charged. It is argued that this would bring additional resources into the NHS, though critics assert that it would lead to a two-tier system with a poorer service being offered to those who had not contracted out. However it is hard to see why this scheme should attract people unless their health insurance policies were made tax-deductible. At a time when attempts are being made to simplify the tax system, and remove as many reliefs as possible, this might be considered a reactionary policy. Moreover, if this scheme was to permit additional funding of the NHS, and not merely provide those who had contracted out with fiscal, and probably medical, privileges, the granting of such tax relief would probably be accompanied by a general raising of tax rates to compensate the Treasury for the money lost. A comparison with the effect of tax relief on mortgages is useful. It has been calculated that if this was abolished, the standard rate of tax could be reduced to 15 pence in the pound.

43.   Few other countries finance their National Health Service as we do. The most common European system is by compulsory insurance. This is generally divided between employer and employee. In some cases it covers all medical treatment; in other countries, such as France, the patient remains responsible for paying for part of it, and it is common to take out private insurance to cover this. There are certain clear advantages in systems based on insurance. The chief one is that the medical services and the patient are brought into a contractual relationship, enforceable in law, and that this exerts a certain discipline which is perhaps absent from the British system.

44.   Nevertheless insurance systems create their own problems, even when they are compulsory. They accentuate the problem of the poor, whose insurance has to be funded or subsidised by the State; and the gradations of poverty make this inevitably invidious. Furthermore there is little evidence that they help to contain costs, and some evidence that they encourage costs to rism. It may be mentioned in passing that comparisons which show that other countries spend a higher proportion of their Gross Domestic

Product on Health than Britain does, do not necessarily demonstrate that they spend money more effectively. It is possible to spend more for the same service, or even for a poorer one.

45.   It does not seem to me that advocates of changing to a system based on insurance have fully appreciated the difficulties that would arise in making such an attempt in a fully-developed country. A long transitional period would certainly be required if only because such a high percentage of NHS patients consists of people who are no longer working, and who could not be expected suddenly to make provision for paying insurance from pensions. It would of course be possible to add a sum to the State retirement pension to cover insurance costs, and for the State to transfer this to insurance companies; but the actuarially-based premium for old people would be extremely high, the cost to the State correspondingly considerable; and it could therefore be twenty years at least before such a system achieved its aims of providing more money for the National Health Service, making that service more efficient, and reducing public expenditure.

46.   Some advocate a system of Health Service vouchers. These would be issued by the State according to a scale which would take age, disabilities and possibly income into account. They would then be invested with insurance companies, or, in some schemes, could be used for direct payments for medical services, or, in others, entrusted to Health Maintenance organisations. Any voucher system has the advantage of introducing a degree of market discipline into the relations between Health Services and patients. It has the disadvantage of introducing far greater uncertainty than now prevails, and probably of accentuating the difference between the treatment received by rich patients, who can top up their vouchers from their own resources, and poor ones who can't.

47.   The virtue of markets is that they increase choice, encourage producers to seek to satisfy consumers, and so make the system responsive to what people want. Their vice is that they always serve the rich better than the poor.

48.   It may well be that the rich and knowledgeable manage to work the NHS better than the poor and ignorant, and therefore to extract better service from it. Yet all systems for financing by insurance or vouchers are likely to be more difficult to understand and more complicated to work, and therefore to make the difference between the best treatment and the poorest wider.

49.   There are two questions about money: how it is raised and how it is spent. It is easier to propound new or different systems of raising money than to suggest more effective ways of spending it, for the latter depends on an exact knowledge of how the NHS actually spends the money it receives. Yet this may well be the most fertile field for investigation and experiment. The weaknesses of the NHS may lie in its structure and administration rather than in the means by which it is financed.

50.   The divorce of revenue from expenditure whih is a feature of the NHS has the advantage of reminding us that no health service can offer value for money because we do not think of health in terms of money. The suggestion that we might be wiser to concentrate on questions of structure and administration is worthwhile it if means that we ask people what they want from the NHS and get, and what they want and don't get; and then consider how we can best secure the former and put right the latter.

VII   The Speakers: Their Arguments and Some Responses

51.   Professor Roy Weir of the University of Aberdeen holds the post of Chief Scientist to the Scottish Office. He spoke on *Options and Constraints*, and if he was guarded on account of his official position, he was less guarded than might have been expected.

52.   He considered these matters under five headings: expenditure, effectiveness, efficiency, equity, and experiment.

53.   There is almost no limit to what might be spent on health care, but at a certain point it might be apparent that the benefit received was low in proportion to the cost. Economists, he observed, told us that services might be usefully expanded till benefits obtained did not exceed the costs incurred. The value of such a principle was that it focused attention not on how much is spent but rather upon what it is spent; one pound spent well might be worth more than two pounds spend badly. To make such a judgement however, systems of calculating costs and evaluating benefits must be improved; meanwhile some measure of rationing was inevitable, 'perhaps even essential'.

54.   To say this, one reflected, was to admit that the delivery of health care was practised in an imperfect world, in which however much we may prefer steak, there are days when we can afford only mince.

55.   Effectiveness and efficiency might be deemed the same thing, but a distinction could be made. Effectiveness was related to the definition of aims, efficiency to their achievement. Such separation of closely related concepts might at least aid clear thinking. The test of effectiveness remained the NHS's loyalty to the principles set out in 1944: the provision of the best medical and other facilities, these to be free at the point of access. There was a need for the various elements in the service to be appraised in this light; 'it would be an act of immense folly to allow further proliferation of a fragmented system which could not be documented or co-ordinated. Evaluating health care and measuring health will become impossible of we do not know why we are doing what, to whom and with what outcome.

56.   With regard to efficiency the practice had been to limit resources available and demand more output, or to reduce resources and demand the same output. There was however another aspect of efficiency which should be taken into account. This was its responsiveness to consumer preference or choice. 'Producing goods at low unit cost which nobody in their right mind would want ought not to be profitable or acceptable.' The difficulty was that patients as consumers lacked information and the knowledge on which to base their choice. They had therefore to delegate this function to doctors who were expected to make wise decisions on their behalf. This situation made many economists uneasy because it meant that decisions on what should be provided, and in what quantity, were made by the provider and not by the consumer.

57.   He did not say, though he might have done, that in this respect health services are like everything else funded by the State. Just as it is the Health Service which determines how much health care should be provided, and of which quality, so it is the Ministry of Transport, and not the motorist, that decides which roads should be built and which improved.

58.   Professor Weir touched the fringe of this question when he asked what there would be to choose even if greater choice were offered. 'If new methods of funding are to be considered should intentional variations in the services be provided to allow meaningful choice?'

59.   This is an interesting suggestion. When you go out to eat, you can choose to go to a pub or a five-star restaurant, and you choose according to your inclination or your purse. Would such choice be acceptable in matters of health care? Could it be reconciled to ideas of equity?

60.   Equity was 'near the top of the objectives of a national health care system.' 'In theoretical terms, to argue for equal treatment for equal need is straighforward; in practical terms of course the measurement of medical need or health status is difficult and subjective.' Moreover it was impossible to have a health service which was both completely equitable and completely efficient.

61.   Professor Weir, of necessity perhaps, couched this observation in abstract language, but it seems to me so important that it ought to be plainly repeated. If there are no waiting-lists and if every hospital has an equal range of up-to-date equipment and highly skilled staff, then that equipment will be unused and that staff unemployed (*though* still paid) part of the time. That is an inefficient use of resources. Conversely, if everyone (or anyone) has to wait for a chance to make use of the services of staff and equipment, that is an inefficient response to need; patients waiting for an operation are not like consumers waiting for a new car—their condition may deteriorate (though Professor McColl later reminded us that waiting-lists could have a therapeutic value: 'patients get healed on waiting-lists') so that the operation becomes more difficult, more dangerous and even more expensive. On the other hand, if a service is fully used, and if the distribution of that service imposes unequal waiting-time on patients, with some having to be awarded priority, not always for medical reasons, any gain in efficiency is made at the expense of equity.

63.   Professor Weir's final E was experiment. Continuous experiment

made evaluation difficult. Yet if any major change was contemplated, it seemed essential that it be preceded by a number of experiments relevant to local conditions. 'By such an approach appropriate options for different parts of the country would evolve.'

63.   The concept of appropriate options for different parts of the country, and the cautious welcome to experiment, signify that a National Health Service need not be a Uniform Health Service.

64.   'The dilemma is that effectiveness, efficiency and equity are all essential parts of an adequate system, but to a degree are in conflict.' 'At the same time we must define the nature and implications of consumer choice'.

65.   This general introduction was followed by(a session entitled 'Public versus Private Financing'. The two speakers were Professor Walter Holland, who is Professor of Community Medicine at St Thomas's Hospital, London, and Professor Alan Maynard, who is Professor of Economics at the University of York. The first has spent all his working life in the NHS; the second's interest in the subject is academic: he has studied the economics of health care as he might have studied the economics of transport. We were therefore offered views of the subject from two very different angles.

66.   Professor Holland observed that any sensible discussion must start by considering what we knew about the need and demand for health services, the use of such services and the result of that use.

67.   This was not easy. Such studies as existed showed wide variation in the use of hospital and general practitioner services between different parts of the country and different social groups. There was no satisfactory general explanation for this.

68.   It seemed that 75 per cent of the patients of a practice might consult their GP in the course of a year. In slightly under half these cases contact was initiated by the doctor. More than a quarter of contacts were concerned with old symptoms, less than a quarter with new ones. The majority of contacts were under the control of those responsible for the delivery of services. Of all contacts about 10 per cent were referred to hospitals as out-patients, and 1 per cent were admitted to hospital. Just under nine cases out of ten therefore stopped at the GP. It was impossible to say whether a low rate of referral was good or bad.

69.   That was, I thought, an observation worth pondering. Clearly a GP who was skilled in diagnosis, or one who was experienced and confident, might handle certain cases which another might refer. That might be good for the patient and cheaper for the Health Service. On the other hand failure to refer might be a sign of ignorance, brusqueness or over-confidence, and might harm the patient and involve the NHS in higher costs at a later date. Once again generalisations about the health service were shown as inadequate because they could not take account of variations in individual skill and matters of personality.

70.   Nevertheless, some things were clear. Major factors in determining whether a case was referred or not were the supply of the service and the certainty doctors had that treatment would be effective: there was far greater variation in referrals for caesarean section than in referrals for acute appendicitis. The only condition for which use, demand and need were all met was pregnancy.

71.   On the other hand there were examples of demand without an effective result. 'Where services are provided because individuals are able to pay for them. inappropriate, ineffective services are often offered. Perhaps the best example of this is multi-phasic screening for the middle-aged'; this 'perk of business-men' produced little benefit, and such checks, if more widely used, could increase NHS costs by as much as 10 per cent with no corresponding benefit. Privately financed systems tended to invest in high technology services, which were expensive and often of little medical benefit.

72.   Again, an analogy presented itself to me: the benefits of eating in expensive restaurants rather than at home are not nutritional.

73.   To spend more on health was not necessarily to spend better. This was borne out by comparisons between the United Kingdom and the United States. There were wide variations in the mortality from conditions such as acute appendicitis, tuberculosis and hernia between different countries, and 'the country that has the best developed privately financed system of care has the worst record in this field.' In a system led by consumer preference things of little use were often introduced. On the other hand a system dominated by medical practitioners themselves might be unresponsive to patients' preferences and emotional needs; 'they would often defend or try to introduce methods of treatment and management that are ineffective.' Ultimately the problem was 'not one of finance, but of the effective use of resources in meeting need and demand.'

74.   Professor Holland spoke as one committed to the NHS, yet puzzled to determine how successful that service is. It is hard to see how this could be otherwise in a system where the majority of patients have no choice but to make what they can of what they are offered. Yet the complexity of the system, and the sheer scale, are obstacles to efficient measurement. How do you evaluate a service which delivers health care to more than 55 million people, but in which every case begins with a conversation between two individuals: the patient and the doctor?

75.   Professor Maynard: 'Every four or five years the NHS is subject to a radical re-appraisal as reformers search for the Holy Grail. The main value of this re-appraisal is the education of politicians.'

76.   As an opening this was both challenging and deflating; it dispelled any notion that Professor Maynard was about to produce the Holy Grail from under a hat.

77.   There was no simple solution, no Holy Grail, and it was generally agreed that we must adhere to the principles of 1944. If we also rejected the notion of throwing more public money into the service as it was organised at present, we were faced with the choice between finding other sources of money, of which the most obvious was the extension of private insurance, or of making better use of existing resources; one way to do this could be the creation of an 'internal market'.

78.   As to the first course, he pointed the contrast between Scotland and the South of England. In Scotland the NHS was better funded—he used the expression 'over-resourced'. There were no waiting-lists [Can this be true?] and there was almost no private market. In the South of England there were about 200 private hospitals, most of them small, with 10,500 beds; there were also 1,300 private beds within the NHS.

79.   There was a discrepancy here which he did not pursue, but it seemed to me that his comparison called into question the statement commonly made that the problems of the NHS could not be solved by more direct investment from the Treasury: for if the perceived problems of the NHS are not so acute in Scotland where more money is spent, mightn't the answer simply be to spend an equivalent amount of money where they are acute? This answer does not of course measure the efficiency with which money is used in Scotland.

80.   The question of measurement is important. Professor Maynard observed that if we had poor evidence about the efficiency of the NHS, we had even less about the private sector. Moreover, leaving that question aside, to extend the private sector by some means of public subsidy would mean the abandonment of the 1944 principles.

81.   He therefore turned to the internal market. There were numerous possible varieties. As an example he offered one in which the Health Board Manager was allocated a budget and made free to spend it where he wished. He would therefore become a trader dealing in different sorts of health care, specialising in the provision of some for his clients, while buying other types on their behalf from other Boards; and of course repeating this process in reverse for the clients of other Boards. In such a system, the doctor would have to act as guardian of the patient's interests; the responsibility for exercising the consumer's choice would be delegated to him.

82.   Such a scheme, he observed, raised several problems. The first was the price of care. How would this be fixed? Then the contractual position of doctors would be changed. Third, such a scheme might reduce even a notional freedom of choice, for patients might find themselves assigned to particular hospitals according to contracts made between those hospitals and the General manager of the Health Board responsible for them. Furthermore the scheme did nothing to resolve the problem of how priorities should be assessed. It might also raise emotional problems and doubts as to the quality of care. Should patients be informed, for instance, about hospital mortality rates, and should they be allowed to choose on the basis of such knowledge?

83.   The importance of this question may be gauged from a table of statistics published in *The Times* on 11 July; this revealed a wide range of variation in hospital mortality rates. Certainly these bare figures would deter some patients from entering particular hospitals. Yet they are a poor guide to performance unless related to a detailed survey of hospitals' admissions policy and of the social circumstances of their clientele. 'A little learning is a dangerous thing', and a smattering of statistical information even more so.

84.   Professor Maynard then introduced the question of 'capital markets'. If an 'internal market' in services was operating, would it not then be logical to permit Health Boards to raise capital? Such permission might let them offer a fuller, but more expensive, service—it would be more expensive because they would have to pay interest on the capital, which is not a requirement placed on capital expenditure under the existing system.

85.   His conclusion was—perhaps surprisingly—conservative. Our lack of information about efficiency and incentives meant that the Holy Grail would certainly not be discovered in the creation of an 'internal market'. We should try to keep ideology in the background while being very clear what our objectives are.

86.   Yet is it possible, I wonder, to form objectives which are free of ideological weighting? Is not ideology in these questions bound to be in the forefront, given that any view of the National Health Service springs either from approval of its principles or from a belief that these principles corrupt its performance?

87.   A discussion followed these papers. I propose to deal with it now simply by listing some of the questions asked, observations advanced, and replies made.

88.   Professor Morag Timbury, Head of the Bacteriology Department at the Royal Infirmary, Glasgow, defined the doctor's dilemma as being 'the interest of patients set against questions of cost and savings'. A doctor was going to manage a budget with the patient's interest uppermost; a budget holder would have a different set of priorities. Professor Maynard agreed that the clinician's freedom to choose would be circumscribed.

89.   Dr Andrew Vallance-Owen, Scottish Secretary of the BMA, asked about the possibility of an internal market with the consultants in charge. This point was not taken up directly at the time, though it would be in Professor McColl's paper delivered in the next session. Professor Holland however observed that there had always been rationing in the Health Service: doctors rationed their time. They were now however being asked to justify the way they did this.

90.   Dr Graham, General manager of the Tayside Health Board, identified two types of Budgeting system. There was the Budget for providing a service, and the Budget for buying care. The first was held by the Health Boards, the second by the patients or their agents, the General Practitioners. [The second seemed to me a hypothetical budget.] He also observed that in Scotland the distinction between public and private services was shadowy, the same people being active in both.

91.   Dr Peter Fisher of the NHS Consultants Association asked whether different styles of treatment were not a necessary part of consumer choice, but Professor Weir doubted its reality, and when the Chairman Sir Alan Peacock asked what evidence we had about consumer choice in the NHS, Professor Maynard remarked that no one looked at the consumer. How, Dr Peter Taylor, Principal Administrative Officer of the National Board for Nursing, Midwifery and Health Visiting, Scotland, asked, would the market apply to patients who were not middle-aged and middle-class? This question, though not closely related to what had gone immediately before, nevertheless had the virtue of drawing attention again to the nub of the matter: poor people need medical attention free at the point of access, and those who would be able to pay generally have little difficulty in working the present system to their own satisfaction.

92.   The title of the second session was: Charging within the National Health Service.

93.   This always arouses strong feeling since it calls the 1944 objectives into question. But the title of the session is of course susceptible to more than one interpretation. There has always been charging within the NHS: there is a charge for labour and a charge for materials. The latter is inescapable, and so is the former unless the service were to be handed over to a Medical Order whose members had taken vows of poverty. The question is not about the existence of charges, but how they are to be settled. This resolves itself into a second question: are they to be charged to patients, either directly or by way of insurance policies, or to taxpayers? One might observe that those pressure groups which favour the costs being borne (that is, the charges being settled) by the taxpayer, include those, the Health Service Unions, who continually urge that labour costs should be higher. Those groups who believe that some costs should be borne by the patient are also generally those who wish to curtail costs in the name of efficiency.

94.   There were two principal speakers: Professor George Teeling Smith, Head of the Office of Health Economics, London, and Professor Ian McColl, Professor of Surgery, Guy's Hospital, London.

95.   Professor Teeling Smith outlined the incompatibilities between economic theory and the principles (and practice) of the NHS. The provision of a 'free service' led to what economists call 'moral hazard'. This means that people tend to consume more than they would if they had to pay for it themselves, or pay for it directly. This behaviour served as a justification for insurance 'co-payments' which would discourage unnecessary use of health services. For the same reason, some element of charging would lead to more economical use of resources.

96.   Yet the objection to this theory had already been identified: 'those most in need are those least able to pay'. Those most likely to be deterred from making demands on the NHS would be those in most need of its services.

97.   Might selective charges, levied in accordance with a means test, be an answer? This would presumably depend on the conditions of the means test. It would be pointless to repeat 'the utter irrationality' of the charge for prescriptions, which was actually paid by only 20 per cent of patients. Nevertheless the imposition of certain charges could bring some useful sums of money into the NHS while also exerting some discipline on demand. It was possible to levy charges fairly, to work out, for example, a fair and satisfactory scheme for imposing 'hotel charges' for the use of hospital beds and for hospital food. The question was however whether, in view of the likely electoral consequences, any government would find such a change worthwhile.

98.   Professor Teeling Smith's exposition of the argument was lucid, too lucid perhaps for some of his audience, who seemed to think his discussion of these matters insensitive. His comparison with the system of financing health services operating in certain European countries, particularly France where co-insurance schemes account for a substantial part of health payments, was too brief to be convincing. He came however to no firm conclusion, but the value of his contribution might be found in his willingness to pose the real question about charging, which is of course its motive. Are charges proposed in order to produce more money for the NHS? Are they proposed to enable Governments to spend less directly on the Health Service and so to reduce taxation? Are they proposed in order to make it possible to use the present resources of the NHS more efficiently?

99.   With Professor McColl we moved away from theory and back to experience. 'The solutions to many of our problems lie in history.' The history of his own hospital had been one of elaboration of structures and expansion of employment which had led to no improvement in standards or output, but to a great increase in costs. A point had been reached in the mid-Seventies when the consultants had been forced to confront this situation and try to rectify matters.

100.   There were two ways of coping with hospital costs of income did not increase to keep pace with them. You could limit the number of people employed, or you could limit the amount of work done by the same number of people. (Limit of course really meant reduce.) A hospital spent its money on staff and on materials, which included all provision for patients. Though 70% of Guy's budget went on salaries, the second course was the easier to adopt. It was simpler to close a ward or perform fewer operations than to dismiss staff or decide not to replace them.

101.   Guy's had responded by introducing a new management structure to control costs. The hospital was put in the charge of a part-time Clinical Unit Director, who reported directly to the District General Manager and was supported by the Chief Executive responsible for all general management of the hospital. He worked in association with the Director of Nursing and was assisted by a central team consisting of the Clinical Superintendent responsible for medical staffing and hospital development, who also chaired the Quality Assurance Committee. The other members of the central team were the Director of Operations responsible for hotel and support services, the Hospital Finance Director and the Personnel Director.

102.   Below this level the hospital was divided into thirteen Clinical Directorates, each headed by a Clinician supported by a Nurse Manager and Business Manager. These directorates were granted as much autonomy as possible in the organisation of work, admission of patients and purchase of materials.

103.   Two principles had been established. First, management accountability was distinct from professional accountability. Second, decentralisation of authority to the Directorates should encourage, and had indeed, encouraged, a sense of responsibility and initiative.

104.   Accordingly in the past three years Guy's had been able to give up 20 per cent of its beds, reduce manpower by 17 per cent (575 posts) and expenditure by almost £8 million per annum (15 per cent of its Budget), and at the same time experience an improvement in productivity. The shedding of superfluous jobs and the encouragement of personal responsibility and initiative had greatly improved morale.

105.   Professor McColl observed that 'although every other department has increased enormously over the past thirty-five years the number of surgeons in the District is the same now as it was in 1951.' Over-manning and restrictive practices were the great enemy of efficiency in the NHS. Decentralisation was an effective response: 'we've got all the ward sisters fascinated by the cost of everything'. Nevertheless it was generally true that, throughout the NHS, you still found restrictive practices at every level.

106.   I suspect that most of the audience found Professor McColl's account of the reforms effected at Guy's by the introduction of clinical budgeting encouraging. It seemed to me an example of intelligent conservatism. Change was admitted, even welcomed, in order that fundamentally the NHS could remain the same.

107.   The ensuing discussion, not surprisingly therefore, concentrated more on the questions raised by Professor Teeling Smith. The dexterity with which he had skated round patches of thinnish ice in his argument aroused some hostile comment. Dr Robert Maxwell, Secretary of the King's Fund Institute, London, observed, however, that it was a mistake to make freedom at the point of use the guiding principle of the NHS; the true principle was equity. There was certainly evidence from the United States that charging could deter demand; the problem was that the effect was inequitable. The poor were deterred from using medical services for which they had to pay, but not the rich.

108.   Dr Marion Hall, Consultant Physician at the Aberdeen Maternity Hospital, remarked that overuse of services was not stopped by charging, but that underuse became very common indeed. (By this, I understood her to mean that the rich used such services more, and the poor less.) Moreover doctors themselves might no longer be willing to accept patients who could only pay minimum charges: most American obstetricians for example did not take Medicare patients.

109.   Dr Hall's observation offered an apt admonition to take into the afternoon session, which was entitled *Financing of Private Services*. It is probably fair to say that this session was already viewed with a disfavour amounting to hostility by a majority of those present. The mood in the hall seemed defensive, and there was an atmosphere of resentment of what was interpreted as an attempt to chip away at the NHS. Nobody there would have described the service as perfect, but most were firmly attached to its principles. Accordingly the two speakers, Dr Eric Blackadder, Governor and Group Director of BUPA, and Dr David Green, Director of the Health Unit, Institute of Economic Affairs, found themselves addressing an unsympathetic audience. Or at least that was my impression.

110.   Dr Blackadder assured us at once that 'the private sector favours a mixed health economy'. Since he went on to say that only 0.7 per cent of GNP was spent on private health care, this prompted the retort: 'it had better, hadn't it?'. He advocated free market competition not only between the private and public sectors, but also within the NHS itself, and also presumably—though he didn't say so—between the different branches of the private sector. Competition within the NHS, and with the private sector, depended on the establishment of some form of 'internal market'; this is clearly difficult to achieve since 'as currently structured, those responsible for running the NHS do not know the actual cost of much that they do, and those who use the service do not appreciate the value of what they receive.'

111.   That observation seemed to be skating on thinnish ice, for Dr Blackadder was no more able (or willing) than anyone else to attempt the difficult task of defining value. No doubt that is a philosophical question, but in so far as a great part of the debate circles round the cost-value equation, it is surely an inescapable one. There are admittedly certain types of elective surgery on which it may be able to place a price-tag which established their value. You can price a nose-straightening operation in much the same way as you can price a new kitchen, and it may be said that in such a case the price represents the perceived value. But how do you do the same thing with heart-bypass surgery, or an operation for acute appendicitis?

112.   Dr Blackadder demonstrated the growth of the private sector. 5.7 million people were now covered by private health insurance. This was 10 per cent of the population. Companies paid 57 per cent of premiums, employees 18 per cent and private individuals 25 per cent. The private sector now performed 15 per cent of all elective surgery and 575,000 operations annually. The NHS earned £67 million from private sector payments, while 28,000 NHS patients were treated in private hospitals under contractual arrangements. [What does this cost the NHS?] Private sector spending was running at between £2.1 and 2.2 billion a year.

113.   This is approximately 10 per cent of NHS spending, and, since many patients insured with the private sector also make use of certain NHS facilities it would seem that those patients are taking more than their fair share of health resources. This may well be misleading, since a great many of those treated within the private sector will be elderly patients, and even within the NHS itself elderly patients receive more than what would be a fair share, calculated on a strictly arithmetical basis, of NHS resources. It must also be remembered of course that those registered with private insurance companies continue to contribute to NHS costs through the taxes they pay, and would make greater demands on the NHS if the private sector was outlawed.

114.   Dr Blackadder affirmed that 'access to health care for all regardless of ability to pay must remain paramount.' No advocate of private medicine could 0say otherwise, and still command a respectful hearing; but the admission does suggest that, whatever reforms are made, private medicine as such, by which is meant health care financed by voluntary contributions, will remain the icing on the cake.

115.   He saw a need to expand the private sector and reduce the distinction between it and the public one. The NHS should continue to carry out functions which it alone could provide (long-term care, accident and emergency treatment and surgery), but it should make full use of the services in which the private sector excels. Among these he listed elective surgery, screening, preventive medicine, and health promotion.

116.   One could see advantages for the private sector in this. It would enable it to expand its services and ensure it a steady flow of income from charges levied on the NHS on behalf of its patients, without putting the private sector to the trouble of recruiting new subscribers. It might moreover enable the private sector to keep inurance premiums down by lowering the unit costs of some of its activities. The advantages to the NHS are however more dubious. Indeed there is no advantage to the Service as such unless the private sector can supply these services more cheaply than the NHS itself could; since, as Professor Maynard had said, we know even less about private sector costs than public sector ones, this must remain a matter of speculation. There might of course be an advantage for the patient if use of private sector services ensured prompter treatment, or more agreeable treatment, but, even if it could be established that this was regularly the case, other aspects of NHS services to the same patients might suffer if the cost of this private treatment was not lower than that which the NHS could provide itself.

117.   Dr Blackadder stressed that 'the patient should be seen as a customer in both services: a customer who has the ultimate sanction of refusing to pay for unsatisfactory service and deciding to take his business elsewhere.'

118.   This was a fine ringing declaration of faith, but it seemed to be taking the notion of medical care as a commodity like any other to its limits, especially as unsatisfactory service may mean that the customer is dead, with no subsequent business to take anywhere.

119.   As for financing of health care services, there were a few possibilities: 1) compulsory National Health Insurance with the ability to opt out partly for those who wish to make private provision; 2) a voucher system for use both in the NHS and the private sector; 3) tax relief on private health subscriptions, especially for the elderly; 4) pre-payment medical services such as membership of Health Maintenance Organisations.

120.   'BUPA,' he said, 'does not want to take over the National Health Service, but would like to see the public taking over the NHS at a local level. We would like to see the NHS being responsible for providing health care, and not for running the largest monopolistic industry in Europe. Funding of the service should be separate from provision of health care. The NHS should be free to provide or purchase all services where the best value for money can be obtained. This could include purchasing clinical services from other health authorites or from the private sector.'

121.   As a statement of the claims of the private sector this was agreeably lacking in ambition. It was not particularly controversial either, since some of his demands are already met. Health Boards do already 'purchase clinical services from other health authorities' (though further development of this is inhibited by a laborious and tardy system of payment) and, as Dr Blackadder had shown, from the private sector too. Nevertheless, if lacking in ambitions, this statement was also tendentious. How, for instance, could, or should, the public take over the NHS at local level? By directly elected health boards? By raising its own finance through local taxation? By other fund-raising activities, some of which are common already?

122.   Moreover, while the NHS may be monopolistic, it is clearly not a monopoly. Dr Blackadder had proved that himself. And, while it is obviously a large nationalised industry, it does (as he demands) provide health care; that is its purpose, its reason for existence, and it is not incompatible with its structure, even though that structure may make it more difficult to provide the best or most satisfactory health care in certain respects.

123.   I was puzzled too by his requirement that funding of the service should be separate from the provision of health care; or rather I was puzzled because Dr Blackadder seemed an unexpected person to make this demand. Weren't we closer to that condition with the NHS functioning as it does at present, when 'those responsible for running it do not know the actual cost of much that they do', than we could even be with a system in which performance was more closely related to price?

124.   Dr David Green is Director of the Health Unit of the Institute of Economic Affairs, which has played such an influential part in re-establishing market principles in the economy as a whole, and which has been very closely associated with the so-called Thatcherite revolution. His doctorate is not a medical one, his field of study being Political Science and Sociology. He has been a Labour councillor and is the author of *Working-Class Patients and the Medical establishment* (1985), and of five books or pamphlets concerning health matters, all published by the IEA. The most recent is *Everyone a Private Patient*, which was the title of the paper he gave to the Conference. This paper was ill-received, and it is fair to say that the fault was his, for it was poorly presented and consisted of passages chosen apparently at random, and therefore incoherently, from his far more persuasive book. Anyone who reads this might still disagree with both his analysis and his conclusions, but would nevertheless have to admit that his argument there is far more worthy of respect than the same argument appeared in his address to the Conference.

125.   Dr Green believes that the NHS suffers from an inherent structural flaw: the absence of a link between demand and budgetary allocation. 'So long as Health services are supplied free at the time of use and financed out of taxes, governments will always find themselves confronting not priced demand but unpriced expectations, uninhibited by contemplation of the other goods and services, like houses and education, which might have been enjoyed instead.'

126.   That there is some truth in this argument is evident. It is curious however that he should have chosen houses and education as examples of the other goods and services which might have been enjoyed instead, since the State education service has been financed in the same way as the NHS, and, like it, meets 'not priced demand but unpriced expectations'; while that phrase might also be used, if more tentatively, to describe the provision of local authority houses for those priced out of the housing market.

127.   He argued that 'for forty years people have been told that the Government will take care of them and meet all their health needs. The reality has always been rationing by waiting-lists and the outright denial of treatment disguised as "clinical judgement". The provision of health care in Britain has therefore suffered from the absence of competition, and paradoxically, the expensive and wasteful NHS, in which there is no satisfactory pricing determinant, has also suffered from "endemic underfunding".'

128.   Consequently, he maintained, 'so long as governments try to finance health care from taxation, they will never be able to meet public expectations', for these will always rise to exceed provision. 'The only way that health care could be an entitlement is by means of a bought-and-paid for private contract, under which the actuarially sound premium was paid by the individual or family in return for a contract of insurance, ultimately enforceable at law.' 'No government,' he said, 'can guarantee a right to a service when the cost is unknown.'

129.   This was one of these fine sweeping generalisations that one generally leaves as unchallenged as the waves of the sea. It hardly stands up to examination, and it evaporates if tested by analogy. The fire and police services are also financed out of taxation, and it would be as sensible to say that the only way in which the arrival of the fire brigade to put out a fire in one's home could be an entitlement would be by means of a bought-and-paid-for private contract etc; it would be as sensible to say this, and, when said, it is seen to be ludicrous. Certainly no government can guarantee a right to a perfect service whether the cost is known or unknown—the police, for instance, fail to solve many crimes—but neither can any system based on private contract. The number of actions brought for medical negligence in the United States is evidence of that. A private contract may ensure that the victim of inadequate health care, or his family, may receive compensation; but compensation is not health care. Finally, the last sentence in the preceding paragraph appears logically flawed. First, it subsumes the individual patient to whom a right pertains in the general cost of the NHS, which is a different matter altogether. Second, it confuses the possession of a right with its exercise, although failure to provide the citizen with the opportunity to exercise his right does not annul that right. Indeed, numerous cases brought against health authorities in the courts testify to the existence of a general contract, or tacit compact, between the citizen and the State; and the agencies of the State have frequently been required to pay compensation for their failure to provide adequate health care. The securing of such compensation may be lengthy, laborious and painful; it may require unusual pertinacity; but the fact that it can be done, and has frequently been done, proves that the right to the service is indeed guaranteed and the agencies of the State can accordingly be penalised for trying to deny it.

130.   Dr Green suggested that 'perhaps the most damaging effect of the NHS promise of "free" health care has been the way it has undermined the capacity of people for self-direction, and spread a child-like dependency on the state.'

131. This can be no more than a matter of opinion, but it is an opinion commonly, and fashionably, proclaimed. It has the charm of being beyond the possibility of proof or disproof. It may be observed however that people, at least equally commonly, remark that they are entitled to health care because they have paid for it. That is to say, common language recognises the existence of the contract the existence of which Dr Green would deny.

132. Even if people imagine the service to be free, as Dr Green thinks they do, it still, as he rightly insists, has to be paid for. He made the valid distinction between 'paying a price' which 'is a disposal of income' and paying a tax which is 'a deduction of income'. The latter, he remarked, 'takes away personal responsibility for deciding how much money will go into health care and curtails personal power to choose the best arrangements for the supply of medical services, thereby impeding competition. He observed that 'a lot of health care is not unlike other consumer goods!'

133. Undoubtedly these are fair points. It is equally fair to state, as he then did, that 'the only realistic alternative to taxation is insurance.'

134. Yet a realistic alternative is not necessarily desirable. This part of his argument provoked two rejoinders.

135. First, there is no guarantee that a system of insurance will in fact put the interests of the insurer first. It may well prefer the interest of the Insurance Company. Anyone who has ever had an old car 'written off' by an insurance company and received in recompense a sum quite inadequate to serve even as a down payment on a replacement will know that the interests of the insurer and the company are not always the same. Furthermore, since doctors, hospitals and health authorities, in such a system, will be bound to take out insurance policies themselves, thereby raising the cost of providing health care, disputes will be frequently settled between insurance companies, to their common satisfaction, and over the head of the insurer, to his dissatisfaction.

136. The second rejoinder is more fundamental. Dr Green's distinction between disposal of income and deduction from income is eminently just; it is also the *raison d'être* of the NHS, which is based on the principle that the rich should pay more and the poor less, and the very poor nothing at all perhaps, for the same service. As soon as this principle is abandoned, it must follow, as surely as night follows day, that those who dispose of more income receive more and better health care, while those who dispose of less or none receive less and worse.

137. Less controversially, he pointed out that 'one of the merits of a market is that events can unfold gradually as lessons are learned from the trial and error of the competitive process.' He talked of 'the evolutionary spirit of the market'. It is undeniable that this exists, and can be a powerful force for improvement.

138. Yet it is surely a mistake to suppose that an evolutionary spirit does not already exist in the Health Service. There is after all an influential market which is already to be found, and this is the market in ideas. The world of medical science is a busy market place in which ideas, theories, hypotheses, new methods of treatment are freely traded, evaluated by experiment and comparison, and adopted sometimes with a zeal which suggests that doctors and administrators are neophiliacs. Far from being the stodgy and complacent thing which its detractors delight in painting, the NHS has been in a state of continuous evolution. There can be few areas of life where intelligent innovation has been more welcome than in medicine.

139.   I give Dr Green's conclusion as he presented it in the synopsis of his paper. 'Greater consumer power could be achieved by leaving the National Health Service more or less intact, thus causing the minimum of disruption, but simultaneously permitting people who are dissatisfied to escape and to claim an age-weighted voucher representing the tax they had paid towards the NHS. People opting out would be required to relinquish their claim to free NHS services and to take out private insurance to the value of the voucher or more, including catastrophe cover. The government would no longer face a commitment to finance an unlimited set of health care services, but would make a fixed annual contribution. People who wanted more services would be free to pay more. The pressures on the NHS will ease as individuals opt out, reducing the extent of the open-ended financial obligation faced by government. No one will be "locked into" the NHS, because at any moment each person will be free to escape by choosing the voucher option. Individuals or families choosing to opt out would not be confined to using private hospitals. They could receive care from NHS hospitals as paying customers, thus altering the balance of power between doctor and patient. Above all, everyone, whether rich or poor, would have the opportunity to become a private patient.'

140.   It must be said that this is a very simplified edition of the argument which Dr Green advances in his book, *Everyone a Private Patient*. Being simplified it appears more cavalier in its disregard of difficulties than his full exposition of the case for this system of vouchers is there. Nevertheless there arre certain gaps and inconsistencies in his argument, which ought to be subject to comment, and certain difficulties, which he seems inclined to ignore.

141.   There is first no means of knowing what the initial cost of this scheme would be. In his book he proposes age-weighted vouchers which, at least on his illustrations, do not in fact 'represent the tax paid towards the NHS', unless it is assumed that everyone of a certain age has contributed exactly the same sum towards NHS costs. This may be an unimportant quibble, and the figures which he gives as an example of the probable value of vouchers represent at least a nod towards certain principles of equity of treatment. But since there is no means of knowing how many people would be attracted to his scheme, there is no means of calculating its initial cost. His calculation of the value of hospital vouchers (he would also offer vouchers for primary care) is based on the actual expenditure per head in 1986 in the NHS hospital service, while the age-weightings arre based on those used by personal pensions plans for insurance policies; but of course expenditure per head is not tthe same as expenditure per patient, and it might happen that a great majority of those who took out vouchers in the early years of the reform made no call on the NHS hospital service, while the majority of those who made such a call took out no vouchers. If that was the case, then the intial cost in terms of public expenditure would be very much higher than the present cost of the NHS, for that would remain almost the same while the cost of issuing these (temporarily) unused vouchers would be added to it.

142.   No doubt this would right itself in time. Then the inconsistencies in his argument would become more apparent. It is hard to understand how the 'government would no longer face a commitment to finance an unlimited set of health care services, but would make a fixed annual contribution', since all those who had declined to take out vouchers and had accordingly remained within the NHS would continue to make the same sort of demands—'unpriced demands' as he calls them—that they do at present. The contribution made in respect of voucher payments might be more or less fixed (though actually it would fluctuate, as some people joined the scheme and others died), but in other respects the position and nature of the NHS would remain unchanged.

143.   The suggestion that patients who receive vouchers and invest them with insurance companies should be able 'to receive care from NHS hospitals as paying customers' might, as he says, alter the balance of power between doctor and patient; it could scarcely fail to create a difference between the treatment given these patients and that accorded those who remained within the NHS. At present, treatment of private patients within the NHS has little effect on standards because there are so few of them. If they came to constitute a sizeable percentage of hospital patients, as they must if his scheme is to work, this would be bound to change. The two-tier system, deplored by all those committed to NHS principles, could not be avoided.

144.   It is a vulgar error to suppose that all those who now use only the NHS are 'locked into it'. The fact is that choice already exists. People who want more services are already free to pay more. 10% of the population do so. A great many others could if they chose, but decide to spend their money on other things. Many parents with children of school age prefer to pay school fees, though a 'free' tax-funded school system is already available, rather than buy additional health insurance. Others prefer holidays or consumer goods. Dr Green's proposals might make choice available to more, but choice already exists and this choice is rejected by many who could afford it.

145.   The voucher system might widen the choice of the sort of health care people would receive, but since the vouchers would have to be spent on health insurance, and since they would still have to be financed out of taxation, it is unlikely that they would afford people any wider choice as to whether they spent this money on health or on something else. To take money in tax, and repay it in the form of vouchers, which could only be paid to an insurance company, seems to offer only an illusory freedom of choice. Moreover, many of those who accepted the voucher might find themselves dismayed by the further sums demanded from insurance companies, especially for the catastrophe cover which Dr Green, if I understand him rightly, would make obligatory.

146.   Finally, Dr Green tells us in his book that 'long-stay provision for the elderly, mentally handicapped, mentally ill and physically disabled' would be 'excluded' from his voucher system, 'because these are "caring" rather than "curing" services which are best provided according to separate principles.'

247.   Expenditure on these groups and on services for them is a principal, and growing, element in NHS spending. Expenditure on people over the age of 75 amounted to 20.4 per cent of NHS expenditure in 1973/4 and 27.5 per cent in 1984/5. Accordingly the voucher scheme ignores the area of spending which is certain to impose ever greater demands on the NHS, unless it was to be contained by providing a poorer standard of service.

148.   So, while this proposed system might hold some attraction for individuals who are dissatisfied with NHS standards and who dislike the denial of choice which they believe they experience in the NHS, it would do nothing to reduce public expenditure (and might increase it) and little to resolve the financial problems of the NHS, despite the fact that it was these problems and the NHS financial structure which gave rise to this debate. To pursue the voucher scheme looks like determined progress up a blind alley.

149.   I have dealt at some length with Dtr Green's paper because he posed the most radical challenge to the NHS. The subsequent discussion offered him little support. The protective mood towards the NHS was most simply encapsulated by Mr W A Smith of the Shetland Islands Council who observed that 'we were being coaxed back into a system that has been tried and failed.'

150.   Professor Kendell, Dean of Medicine, University of Edinburgh, made the point that the private sector did not in fact bear all its own costs. The NHS trained its own staff, and those who worked in the private sector too; elective surgery operations in the private sector were frequently performed with the help of NHS nurses. The true cost of the health care provided by the private sector was therefore not reflected in the insurance premiums charged.

151.   This view received some support from Professor David Vines, Adam Smith Professor of Political Economy, University of Glasgow. He suggested that if people joined a private insurance scheme they should lose their NHS rights. This would presumably result in higher premiums since BUPA or any other insurers would then have to offer comprehensive health care. He suggested, more tentatively, that they might receive tax rebates; it is unlikely however that such a rebate would amount to the cost of comprehensive health insurance.

152.   Professor Vines returned the argument to the question of charges. If pitched at the right level, these reduced demand. Unfortunately, they reduced both unnecessary demand, which might be desirable, and necessary demand, which was inequitable. All private health systems involved some system of insurance, and the effect of insurance was to remove inhibitions on demand. There was therefore no reason to suppose that an insurance-based system could cut overuse. On the other hand some element of supply-side charging might offer benefits.

153.   Mr J A Rennie, of the Scottish Home and Health Department, brought up the problem of capital expenditure. How would this be provided if the concept of a centrally funded NHS was abandoned? If there was no central planning of capital development, it was hard to see how this would correspond to need. Professor Teeling Smith agreed that all over Europe there was central capital planning, no matter how health services were financed.

154.   It seemed to me that in raising this question Mr Rennie, no doubt as a result of his experience, exaggerated the difficulties: many businesses of great size, multi-nationals for example, seem able to plan capital expenditure to their own satisfaction in response to perceived needs; so of course do the BUPA hospitals. Nevertheless, it is quite likely that a health service which operated purely in the private sector would fail to supply the hospital needs of everybody; it would always be more attractive to build hospitals for the rich than for the poor.

155.   Professor Michael Oliver, President of the Royal College of Physicians, Edinburgh, observed that the Chief Scientist to the Scottish office had begun by talking of demands being greater than resources. No one had disputed this. Yet it was important to be clear as to just what we meant by the word 'demands' in this context. Were we talking about consumer choice, or about the provider of the service asking for what he thought necessary? They were not the same thing. Nor was it right to say that a shortfall should be deplored in every case. There was for instance enormous pressure from pharmaceutical companies on doctors to prescribe more drugs, and on patients to demand them; in the USA for instance a cartel of three Drug Companies had clubbed together to tell the American public about their blood-cholesterol level, and so persuade them to buy corrective drugs. This was an example of induced and unnecessary demand.

156.   The private sector appeared to him to be of value on the fringes of Health Care. He couldn't see that it would take much off the public sector in acute cases or indeed in the diagnostic sector.

157.   A profession could become complacent, but professional standards of conduct were best maintained by a profession's own regulatory body. The Royal Colleges were very concerned with the maintenance of standards.

VIII   Reflections

158.   Few intellectual activities are more agreeable than criticism of the status quo, and the elaboration of an alternative system. Whoever indulges in such activities is able to contrast the real with the ideal, and it is no wonder if the former comes off worse. The National Health Service is well-established. Its flaws and failures are patent. It can be examined, dissected, and reproved. This cannot be done with any alternative system. Advocates of reform are fond of comparing the NHS with other systems in other countries, and there is some merit in this. Yet the comparison can never be exact, for these systems are the product and reflection of the history, social structure and culture of those countries, as the NHS is of ours. Even a straightforward comparison of spending on health in different countries may be misleading; 'there is strong evidence that much of the explanation for national difference in health spending lies in differences in national wealth' (Maxwell: BMJ, 21 May 1988.)

159.   It was asserted earlier that we would not have created a service like the NHS if we had been creating a health service from nothing. That in itself was an admission of the compelling force of what actually is. In like manner, any proposed reform of the NHS has to start with the NHS as it actually is. We have a very fully developed system of providing health care. Its financing is simple, and a great many of its patients have been contributing to that financing through the taxes they have paid for the whole of the life of the NHS. They feel it is their service even when it treats them badly, and the majority have no wish to pay for it in any other way. Nor do they wish to see the providers of health care discriminating between patients according to their ability to pay.

160.   In general, few in the medical profession wish to see radical reform. The strength of the profession's loyalty to the NHS is the service's most valuable asset, and it should not be dismissed as evidence merely of professional conservatism. Moreover, it is both impertinent and stupid to suggest that the profession is attached to the NHS because it is a providers' service from which they do very well. It may indeed be a providers' service, and if so this may be one of its flaws, but it is probable that most members of the medical profession would do very much better if the NHS was financed in another fashion. Their attachment to the service cannot be divorced from their belief that financing health care from taxation is the most equitable manner of enabling them to fulfil their professional obligations.

161.   Opposition to the present method of financing health services in this country comes principally from economists and ideologues. (The two categories may overlap.) These critics range from the respectable to the ridiculous. We may ignore the latter, saying with Burke that 'they have no respect for the wisdom of others; but they pay it off by a very full measure of confidence in their own. With them it is a sufficient motive to destroy an old scheme of things, because it is an old one. As to the new, they are in no sort of fear with regard to the duration of a building run up in haste; because duration is no object to those who think little or nothing has been done before their time, and who place all their hopes in discovery. They conceive, very systematically, that all things which give perpetuity are mischievous, and therefore they are at inexpiable war with all establishments.' Such are those who would reform the Health Service simply because it is national and they cannot conceive that any good can come from the State; and those who would reconstruct it simply because it is not a market, or rather not one of the type which they recognise, in which the only token of exchange is cash. Their views may be disregarded because they are essentially worthless.

162.   Respectable critics may however be properly disturbed by the removal of the NHS from the market place and the ever more evident consequences of that removal. These they identify as the lack of connection between demand and provision, and the tendency towards monopoly with its concomitant vices, which are: waste, the growth of a parasitical bureaucracy and the the proliferation of superfluous jobs; the concentration of decision in the hands of the providers and the consequent indifference to the wants of the consumer. All such vices feed on themselves; a monopolistic body will be seen to develop a greater tenderness for the interests of its own members than for those of the public, until eventually it may exist only to service itself, in perfect indifference to those it was established to serve.

163.   It would be ridiculous to assert that the NHS was in this condition, but false to pretend that these tendencies are not visible. It is indeed their visibility which has persuaded many by nature friendly to the NHS that it is in need of reform.

164.   It is natural first to propose a reform in the method of financing health care, and to look at the examples of other countries. The only practical alternative is a system of insurance-based financing, and Dr Green's system of Health Service vouchers is only a variant of this, intended to offer a freedom of choice to the poor as well as the rich; though, as I have suggested, the intention is not met and the freedom might well be illusory.

165.   The merit of the insurance-based system is clearly first that it establishes a direct link between the service provided and the price paid; and, second, that it may offer the patient a choice of treatment which he does not have under the present system.

166.   It does not necessarily control costs, though it is arguable that the creation of bodies like the American Health Maintenance Organisations may help to do so by improving the bargaining power of consumers. I say this is arguable, for such improvement may only be temporary till the market adjusts itself to take account of the power of such organisations.

167.   It is also arguable whether the individual patient's freedom of choice is greatly enhanced in such a system. In theory no doubt it is, but in practice it seems that it is likely to be curtailed either by the Insurance Company or by the Health Maintenance Organisation which acts as his nominal representative.

168. The analogy with the position of a member of a trade union is perhaps relevant. The trade union will secure some benefits for its members, but in doing so it will deny its members the freedom to negotiate their individual conditions of employment. The trade union may even come to exercise a monopolistic power on its own behalf, and the trade unionist may find that the independence he thought had been secured from his employer has in fact been surrendered to his protector, the Union.

169. This is a variant of the criticism that Professor Maynard levelled at the 'internal market': that the patient might find his choice restricted as he was locked into a contract entered into by two bodies, one acting on his behalf but without his knowledge.

170. But the real objection to a move to a system of insurance-based financing is quite different, and even more formidable. It is not that such a system cannot work effectively, for the experience of other countries shows that it can work quite as well as our system. In some indeed it may work better, though in others perhaps worse. The effectiveness of the system in other countries is not the point. The point is that we are too late to adopt it.

171. All systems of national health care started from a narrow base and developed gradually. All began by providing care for only a minority of the population. The German system, for instance, which is based on compulsory insurance through sickness funds, is more than a hundred years old. It was introduced by Bismarck and it began in a small way with many people excluded from insurance cover. It was, that is to say, the undeveloped product of an undeveloped state with an undeveloped economy. It was more advanced than contemporary systems of health care provided by Britain and other European countries, but it was primitive in comparison with what even an undeveloped European country like Greece or Portugal offers today. Any undeveloped country may choose between adopting an insurance-based or tax-funded system of Health Care, but to move from one to the other in a developed country would be an undertaking of very great difficulty.

172. Even if such a switch was achieved—and it would probably have to be spread over a long period of transition—it would long be perceived as inequitable. Those who had contributed to the NHS through taxation would feel cheated if now compelled to take out insurance cover, even if this was provided by the State by means of tax credits. There is for instance a firm belief among older people who use the service most, that they have already paid their fair share during their working life. Along with this goes the agreeable conviction that at present the rich contribute more and get the same treatment; it would be hard to disabuse people of the notion that a switch to insurance would mean that those who paid most were treated best. After all, that is precisely the position in the United States.

173. In short, while a switch to an insurance-based system might do something to correct the balance between demand and resources, it would he hard to sell the idea to the electorate who would view it with suspicion and resentment. Moreover it is not certain that it would correct that balance.

174.   Ultimately there is little to be said for a reform which would find favour with neither the medical profession nor the public.

175.   The principal value of this Conference seemed to me to be this; it established that all those who approach the problems of providing health care from the starting-point of how it should be financed are starting from the wrong place. The question is not how money should be raised, but how it should be spent. A great deal of work has been done on this immense question with its endless ramifications, which it would be impossible to summarise here. I shall however approach the subject, albeit briefly, from two angles.

176.   In some cases the provision of health care may be improved by spending less money; in others it is necessary to spend more. That should suggest that it is not simply a question of money. It has of course often been pointed out that the easiest way to save money is to provide less health care. As Robert Maxwell put it in that BMJ article I have already quoted: 'the easiest way for any NHS hospital to balance its books is to do less clinical work or to reduce standards.' Nobody, I presume, finds this satisfactory.

177.   Nevertheless Professor McColl's account of reforms at Guy's Hospital appeared to me cogent testimony that economy and medical excellence can be complementary. The separation of responsibility for hospital administration and clinical work on the other hand seems a recipe for inappropriate economy and a low standard of medicine. Nobody would wish consultants to be swamped by administrative work, but if they are not involved in decisions as to have money should be spent, they have no incentive to practice economy; conversely, if they are excluded from administrative matters, questions of staffing for instance, administrative costs will almost certainly rise at the expense of clinical work. To give hospitals back to the consultants would be a worthwhile reform, and to make hospitals self-governing another.

178.   A self-governing hospital should be free to raise extra revenue, as it can, without penalty. Partly for this reason, and partly for the wider benefits that would accrue, the boards of governors and hospital management committees which were disbanded in 1974 should be revived. Sir Robert Bayliss, assistant director, research unit, Royal College of Physicians, London, has written: 'both had done much to interest the community in *their* hospital. Such bodies were perhaps an anachronism, but much that is good in British public life is anachronistic. Our board members were astute, outstanding people from many walks of life who gave their services free. We lost for example the wise counsel of the chairman of ICI.' At the very least the introduction of governors who are neither medical professionals nor bureaucrats admits local public opinion to a share in the management of a hospital.

179.   If hospitals are self-governing, some sort of 'internal market' and some sort of trading relationship with the private sector is likely to develop naturally, where it is seen to be of advantage. A degree of specialisation in clinical work in different hospitals leads both to economical and efficient use of resources and to greater expertise. A surgeon who performs a particular operation twice a week is likely to be more adept than one who performs it six times a year.

180. While it would be possible for hospitals to send bills directly to central government for work performed above the block grant which they might receive for staffing and administrative costs, it probably makes sense to keep regional health authorities in being, and for them to become, as it were, holding companies, whose principal function would be the transmission of funds from central government to local agencies, and the supervision of work and maintenance of standards.

181. The regional health authorities, by whatever name they were to be known, could also co-operate usefully with the department of Health, the Scottish Office and the Northern Irish Office, in planning capital expenditure. This should however be more receptive to evidence of what the public wants than it is now. At present capital expenditure is determined by what the Government and its agencies think the people need; it pays little attention to what they say they want. Its criteria are those which will enable services to be 'efficiently' provided rather than those which would provide services that most effectively—to employ Professor Weir's distinction—responded to what people manifestly want. A policy of centralising services is pursued because this is perceived to be the most efficient means of providing them, even though this means that in important, if unquantifiable, respects the service then provided is less satisfactory to patients and their families than a locally-provided one would be. Nowhere is this more apparent than in the provision of maternity services.

182. In this context it may be observed that much talk of 'consumer choice' is misleading. A patient rarely chooses, or could be in a position to choose, between two different forms of treatment as he or she might choose between different brands of washing-machines. In many cases only one form of treatment is appropriate; in others the patient does not have the knowledge that would be necessary to make such a choice, and could not indeed acquire it. One may remark in passing that in other areas of the market such choice as exists is often illusory. In buying a washing-machine we are often guided by the salesman's assurances that A is better than B, or we decide to buy B because we cannot afford A; I do not think we would any of us regard it as a satisfactory exercise of consumer choice if we felt compelled to decide on a certain operation because it was cheaper than another. No doubt such a decision is sometimes made over our heads (as it is made also in insurance-based systems), but the real denial of consumer choice in the NHS is frequently social rather than individual; a hospital, for instance, is closed, or has certain facilities withdrawn from it, because such closure or withdrawal fits into public expenditure plans, and this is done even though the local community is generally hostile to the action. It would be more reasonable, and responsive to public opinion, if instead people were told that their local hospital could only be funded to a certain level, and, that if they wished it to remain in being, they must be prepared to find additional money from some other source.

183. The principal causes of public dissatisfaction with the NHS are the length of waiting lists, the uncertainty bred by them, and the conviction that hospitals are organised for the convenience of those who work in them rather than those whom they exist to serve. These are maqtters where improvement is possible even within the present structures of the NHS; but improvement would be easier if a measure of decentralisation took place. Waiting-lists are inevitable in any system which is not operating with considerable unused excess capacity; they are made intolerable by poor liaison, uncertainty and discourtesy. Most people would accept being put on a waiting-list for non-acute surgery if they were given a date, some time in advance, on which they would be treated; and if they were confident that the hospital would adhere to that arrangement. Poor liaison and poor time-keeping are evidence of indifference to the patient as a person; it should be noted that General Practitioners, who in effect act as patients' agents in these matters, are frequently treated with similar discourtesy; they too find it hard, sometimes impossible, to discover what hospitals plan for their patients.

184.   Much of the discussion about the NHS centres on hospitals, but perhaps the Service's worst fault is its misuse of what should be its most important members, the General Practitioners. Their role has been diminished since the inception of the NHS and medicine has suffered as a result. The following paragraph is taken from an article in *The Spectator* of 23 July, 1988.

185.   'The Treasury still considers the purpose of the GP is to ration access to hospital care, not replace it with his own. The British general practitioner is largely excluded from the demanding business of looking after the really sick. He must be content to receive out of date letters about patients treated in hospitals in which he has no visiting rights, with instruments and drugs which he may well have difficulty in recognising. Certainly in the inner cities, close to the large teaching hospitals, the GP's world is, as Mrs Edwina Currie recently said, one of stamp-licking, amateur psychotherapy and repeat prescriptions. Outside the cities there is marginally more for the GP to do, but the restrictions imposed on him by the NHS represent a dreadful waste of talent.'

186.   I believe this is generally true. The author, Myles Harris, might have added the final touch of irony: the GP is simultaneously overworked and under-employed. He is often highly valued by his patients, but his value to them is less than it might be.

187.   There are two ways in which better use might be made of GP's. First, instead of closing cottage hospitals and concentrating services in General Hospitals, more cottage hospitals should be built, and some which have been closed should be re-opened. These hospitals should be the responsibility of GP's. Many at present treated in General Hospitals could be cared for more effectively in cottage hospitals by their own doctor and his partners. Such hospitals can, and should, provide maternity services; they can care best for convalescent cases, for non-acute geriatric cases, for those conditions which require nursing rather than surgery, and for those cases, described as terminal, where there is no hope of recovery, and a patient's principal interest is to be allowed to die with dignity with members of his or her family and friends close at hand. Because they are in touch with the local community, they can also provide temporary beds for patients normally cared for at home, whose carers need a holiday. They can provide treatment for minor casualties as well as the casualty departments of large hospitals, and generally very much more conveniently. They have the great merit of being responsive to the needs of local people, and they have been shown to be extremely cost-effective.

188. In the cities where there may be less need of such hospitals (though a number of practices might with advantage join together to operate one), GPs should be granted their own wards in General Hospitals and they 0should everywhere be guaranteed visiting rights to their patients in acute wards. It might indeed be worthwhile for General Practitioner Group Practices to receive extra money which would enable them to take an another partner with responsibility for hospital work, or whose recruitment would allow them to distribute that work among all members of the partnership without impairing their performance of their present duties.

189. Indeed, if those responsible for the administration of the NHS are seriously concerned to remove causes of justifiable dissatisfaction with the service, and so merit the high regard in which it is still held by most people, an enhancement of the role of the General Practitioner is an obvious course of desirable action. The GP is the patient's first link with the service and his most important; but in too many cases that link is, in effect, snapped when the patient enters hospital, and the importance of the GP is consequently devalued.

190. Twenty years ago the Czech leader Alexander Dubcek tried to offer his people 'Socialism with a human face'. It is the fault of the NHS that its human face is too often obscured. Medicine is a human science, but the provision of health care is too often inhumane. All the vices of the NHS stem from its inhumanity. It has therefore taken on the marks of bureaucracy: waste of every kind, extravagance and indifference to human values; it has done this despite the personal humanity and high principles of doctors, nurses and other NHS staff. They are its victims too.

191. It would be absurd of me to presume to offer a plan for its reform. However, this Conference and the reading which I have done have convinced me that the problem does not rest in the manner in which the NHS is financed. I see no reason to believe that a switch from a tax-based to an insurance or insurance-cum-voucher system would effect substantial improvement in the provision of health care, and I am sure that such a change would result in a long period of disruption and bitterness during which the standard of care provided actually deteriorated. It is obviously necessary that we devise better means of measuring the effectiveness and efficiency of what is done within the NHS, but I would suggest that a reform of its structures is the first desirable step.

192. In Paragraph 121 I questioned Dr Blackadder's demand that the public should take over the NHS at a local level; somewhat mockingly. I do not see how that would be possible. Nevertheless, Dr Blackadder's demand, however vaguely expressed and inadequately developed, does seem to me to point in the right direction. Precisely because the NHS is such a huge organization, it is desirable to fragment it, to give the maximum autonomy to each unit, and encourage the taking of decisions and the assumption of responsibility at local level. I believe this can best be done by making hospitals self-governing, while involving non-professionals in their supervision, and by enhancing the role of GP's and encouraging them, indeed making it possible for them, to practise medicine in the full sense of the word whenever possible.

193.   Such devolution of authority and responsibility is in accordance with modern business pracice and theory, and, if I may be permitted a final analogy, it is the way of armies also. In earlier stages of warfare armies generally operated in large units, because their training did not permit them to manoeuvre otherwise. But any student of military history knows that the tendency of an efficient and effective army has been towards the formation of small units capable of operating on their own, and acting on personal initiative.

194.   It is a truism that the NHS is still highly regarded by the public in general. It is easy to pass over truisms, but it should not be forgotten that they are truisms because they are true. That is the first asset of the NHS, and its second is the devotion it inspires in the medical profession. I hope I have managed to show that this is not primarily because they benefit from it themselves—for examination of other systems demonstrates that on the whole doctors and nurses can do very much better for themselves in a cash market; but rather because they believe in the principle that health care should be provided free at the point of access. It would be folly to cast aside, or to imperil, the common devotion to the NHS of the public and the medical profession. But on the other hand it is equal folly to pretend that all is well with the service. It is necessary therefore to look at its weak points and repair them, to consider how it wastes resources, not only of money and material, but of men and women, and in some cases of good-will, and how it might learn not to waste them. I hope at the least I have elucidated some of the arguments and suggested a few directions that might be followed.

THE SPEAKERS

Professor Roy Weir, Chief Scientist, The Scottish Office.

Professor Walter Holland, Professor of Community Medicine, St Thomas's Hospital, London.

Professor Alan Maynard, Professor of Economics, University of York.

Professor George Teeling Smith, Head of the Office of Health Economics, London.

Professor Ian McColl, Professor of Surgery, Guy's Hospital, London.

Dr Eric Blackadder, Governor and Group Medical Director, BUPA.

Dr David Green, Director of The Health Unit, Institute of Economic Affairs, London.

THE DISCUSSANTS

Dr R C Graham, General Manager, Tayside Health Board, Dundee.

Miss Anne Jarvie, Unit Nurse, Greater Glasgow Health Board.

Dr Robert J Maxwell, Secretary, King's Fund Institute, London.

Mr Graeme S Millar, Vice-Chairman, The Pharmaceutical General Council (Scotland).

Professor Morag Timbury, Head of Bacteriology Department, Royal Infirmary, Glasgow.

Dr Andrew Vallance-Owen, Scottish Secretary, The British Medical Association, Edinburgh.

Sir Gerald Elliot and **Professor Sir Alan Peacock**, respectively the Chairman of the Trustees and the Executive Director of The David Hume Institute took turns in chairing the discussion sessions. **Professor Michael Oliver**, President of the Royal College of Physicians, Edinburgh, summed up the day's proceedings.

The Conference Organiser was **Mr H L Snaith**, a Trustee of The David Hume Institute.

THE DAVID HUME INSTITUTE

The David Hume Institute was established as a company limited by guarantee in January 1985, and it is registered as a charity. Its registration number in Scotland is 91239.

The objects of the Institute are to promote discourse and research on the economic and legal aspects of public policy questions.

Honorary President (1988–1991) Judge Thijmen Koopmans, Court of Justice of the European Communities

Chairman Sir Gerald Elliot FRSE

Executive Director Professor Sir Ian Peacock FBA

Secretary and Treasurer H L Snaith

Registered Office, 10 Hope Street, Charlotte Square,
Edinburgh EH2 4DD
Tel: 031 225 6298

HUME PAPERS

1   Banking Deregulation *Michael Fry*
2   Reviewing Industrial Aid Programmes: (1) The Invergordan Smelter Case, *Alex Scott* and *Margaret Cuthbert*
3   Sex at Work: Equal Pay and the 'Comparable Worth' Controversy *Peter Sloane*
4   The European Communities Common Fisheries Policy: A Critique, *Antony W Dnes*
5   The Privatisation of Defence Supplies *Gavin Kennedy*
6   The Political Economy of Tax Evasion *David J Pyle*
7   Monopolies, Mergers and Restrictive Practices: UK Competition Policy 1948–87 *E Victor Morgan*

Published by **Aberdeen University Press**

8   The Small Entrepreneurial Firm *Gavin C Reid* and *Lowell R Jacobsen*
9   How Should Health Services be Financed? *Allan Massie*
10   Strategies for Higher Education – The Alternative White Paper *John Barnes* and *Nicholas Barr*